CORE*Walking*

I0423190

Sciatica / Piriformis Syndrome

Learn to understand the feeling and healing of your pain!

Jonathan FitzGordon

Other books in this series:
Psoas Release Party!
The Exercises of CoreWalking
An Introduction to The Spine

Although every effort has been made to provide an accurate description of posture remedies and their benefits, the information contained herein is not intended to be a substitute for professional medical advice, diagnosis or treatment in any manner.

Always consult your physician or health care professional before performing any new exercise, exercise technique particularly if you are pregnant, nursing, elderly, or if you have any chronic or recurring conditions.

The authors are not responsible or liable for any injuries occurred by performing any of the exercises given or diagnosis made by a user based on the information shown within this document.

TABLE OF CONTENTS

INTRODUCTION

You shouldn't live with pain. Because living with pain it is not really living. It's not living to your fullest. Often we get little pains and think, "Oh, I'll deal with it later." But when your car gets a flat tire, you get it fixed or it's not going anywhere. How about your one and only body? It deserves that kind of constant tuning up. This book will help tune up your body by providing information and tools to address the pain and debilitation of sciatica and piriformis syndrome…and perhaps prevent you or your loved ones from ever dealing with either.

We will give you an in depth look at all of the actors in the drama – your bones and muscles, the sciatic nerve, the piriformis muscle as well as the psoas, your spine and pelvis. We'll look at how they are supposed to work and why they might not be working well. We'll explore how the body operates from conditioned patterns and how these patterns limit our physical potential. Of course, we'll also provide tools and exercises for relief.

However, this book is for more than those who have sciatica or piriformis syndrome. This book is for those who want to understand more about how the body works, those who have grown up around individuals with sciatica and piriformis syndrome and don't want to inherit these issues, and those who don't want to pass them on to their children. As we'll discus, much of our movement is learned behavior from those who raised us. Think about it – often many members of a family will say they have a bad back and the problem is inherited. Yet, what might be inherited is not a "bad" back but rather the movement patterns that lead to pain in the back. So the conditioned patterns that we develop during childhood and bring to adulthood are going to determine the quality of our lives. Your ability to understand and change those patterns determines what kind of body you have. Knowledge of how the body works can help us break cycles of debilitation and pain for ourselves and those we love.

You can change they way your body operates. We all deserve to understand how our body works and how we can work it with it. You can choose to be conscious and to make changes over and over again to be your own healer. You can mindfully create new patterns in your body that allow it to be the beautifully operating piece of machinery and miracle that it is. You can choose to fully live your life.

CHAPTER ONE – SOME BODY BASICS

We'll begin our exploration with how the body works in terms of the muscular-skeletal system – your muscles and your bones. Then we'll examine what the body's structure has to do with sciatica and how we might find ourselves with sciatica.

HOW DOES THE BODY WORK?

Think about Pinocchio hanging from his strings. We're actually a step above our man Pinocchio in that our skeletal structure can hold us upright. Pinocchio moves when the puppeteer pulls on his strings. We move when our nerves tell our muscles to move our bones. Our bones hold us up and our muscles move us, and our nervous system communicates this action. If this system is working properly, then our joints can stay loose, fluid and free, much like Pinocchio's. However, if our bones, nerves, and muscles aren't talking well to each other, we put strain on our precious (and expensive) joints like the vertebrae of the lower back.

The muscular-skeletal system is an amazing piece of machinery. If your body is stacked correctly (one bone on top of the other, one joint sitting well into the next), your bones, the skeletal system itself, can simply hold you up. Of course, the muscles do have some work to do. They need to be properly toned to keep the bones well aligned in this stacking. But let's define what muscle "tone" is. We think of toned muscles as big, buff biceps and rock hard abs. Actually, tone is the base level of engagement of your muscle. Even when your muscle isn't engaged, it still has a certain shape. That's tone. You don't need huge, contracted muscles for good skeletal (bone) alignment. Rather, you need muscles that are strong enough to do what you're asking of them in helping the bones stack.

One reason our muscles lose tone (i.e., become weak) is because we aren't stacking ourselves properly to begin with. We sit in our joints, making some muscles work too hard and others not work at all. The muscles work in pairs, and these pairs work in a reciprocal fashion. When one engages (shortens) its opposite can stretch (lengthen). For example, let's consider the opposites of the hamstring (the muscle at the back of the thigh) and the quadriceps (the muscle at the front of the thigh). When the quadriceps engages, then the hamstring stretches. Give it a try. Lift your knee in the air to the height of your pelvis. Put one hand on your quadriceps (the top) and extend the leg. You should feel it engage or harden. Now do the same motion but place your hand at the back of your leg.

You'll fee your hamstring extend and stretch. This muscle balance is going on throughout the body. So when we aren't using our muscles properly (or at all) then one muscle will get overworked (tighter) and at the same time its opposite will grow weaker (lacking tone). Ida Rolf, the creator of Rolfing and a hero of mine, once said, "People always talk to me about strength or how strong they are, but I always tell them that strength is meaningless, balance is power."

Not stacking our bones properly leads to muscle imbalance, which then prevents us from stacking our bones properly. It all gets very chicken and the egg – what problem came first?! The simple fact is that we are meant to have toned muscles and correct skeletal alignment, and they influence each other.

Moreover, the muscle tone and skeletal alignment impact our nervous system. You can't send a clear, quick message along telephone wires if the poles are fallen down. Similarly, the alignment of the bones determines the freedom of the nerve pathway. Remember the nerves tell the muscles how to move. When you don't have good muscle tone and bone alignment, then the nervous energy of the body is restricted. This means the nerves depend on muscle tone so that they can communicate with those very muscles. Now we're really getting chicken and the egg – we need everything to be working for everything to be working!

Our posture is one of the places we often fall into troubles with our bones, muscles and nerves; in particular, muscular imbalance shows itself in posture. We'll address posture in more detail later in the book. For now, it's important to understand that many of us are not stacked properly. We tend to be short in the back and long in the front. The muscles of our legs, lower back, and neck tend to be short and tight. Does it feel like that in your body? Tightness when you bend over? Tension in the neck? Only the upper back tends to be loose because of tightness across our chest. This short and tight back body comes from the way we stand. Take a look at the diagrams below. Most of us feel like we're standing like the one on the left. Unfortunately, we tend to stand like the one on the right. We tuck our pelvis, which pulls down the lower back and forces the femur (big thigh bone) forward. Movement in one part of the body is always reciprocated in another part. So the tucking of the pelvis may lead to hyperextension of the knees (locking the knees backward past the straight line) and kyphosis (rounding) of the upper back, and also a forward thrust of the head.

Check yourself out in the mirror. Overexaggerate

the stance, but then see if you're doing something like this diagram on the right. Seeing yourself clearly and honestly is a big part of healing and healthy living. Try to catch your reflection while you're waiting on a street corner. Check out the people around you. You'll start to see that short in the back and long in the front is a very common stance.

But don't beat yourself up if you're doing it. Like so many things, our culture has an aesthetic or habit that is actually far from what is natural or good for us. From the time we are little, people tell us to throw our shoulders back thinking this will make for good posture. Look at mannequins or models in advertisements thrusting the pelvis forward to perhaps look thinner. What about our furniture? As couches and chairs get softer and deeper, we spend a lot of time sinking into ourselves instead of maintaining good bone alignment and the muscle tone to hold ourselves up. These messages and patterns affect how we carry ourselves. Essentially we're falling down into our posture instead of standing up. In a way, we are devolving in our physical posture. We are losing the ability to stand up with dignity and fully embody ourselves as humans.

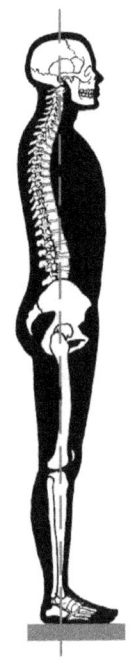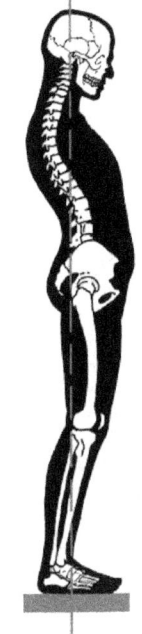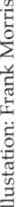

Illustation: Frank Morris

WHAT DOES THIS HAVE TO DO WITH SCIATICA?

Beyond the psychological affects of sinking down instead of standing up, there are a series of chronic pain issues confronting modern man due to this poor posture, poor muscle tone, poor bony alignment, etc. Sciatica and piriformis syndrome are amongst the most common. There are actually two different issues at play here. Sciatica is a bony alignment issue. Something, like a slipped disc, is pressing on the sciatic nerve sending pain down through the leg and sometimes all the way to the foot. This is a nerve injury. With piriformis syndrome, the piriformis is in spasm and it pushes on the sciatic nerve, which passes right under it. You also get that sciatica type pain with piriformis syndrome. Often people aren't sure of the reason for their sciatic pain. In general, the issue of shortness in the back body (the bad posture we saw in that diagram above) contributes to both sciatica and/or piriformis syndrome. Generally speaking, space equals health. So when we're short in the back body, we're compromising the space there. This creates a cramped and then painful environment for the sciatic nerve.

WHY WOULD WE GET SCIATICA?

In the case of something pressing on the sciatic nerve, most often it is a slipped or herniated disc. We're talking about the discs that live in between the vertebrae of the spine, often referred to as intervertebral discs. These discs slip and degenerate for all different reasons. First of all, genetics and imitation play a role. So a family can truly have a bad back issue through many generations where the integrity of the spine is compromised. Discs also become damaged because of trauma. There's the trauma of an acute injury, like a car accident. There's also extended emotional trauma. Our bodies remember everything, and we store tension in our muscles. A history of emotional trauma is going to affect the physical structure of the body. As mentioned, our posture can contribute to poor bone alignment and poor muscle tone, both of which can lead to slipped discs. Finally, diet and nutrition also a play a role in the development of our bodies, and health of the spine.

You could also be experiencing sciatica from a bone pressing into the sciatic nerve. Certain conditions that we'll discuss later can lead to degeneration of the spine that may result in bone pressing onto the spinal column or the root of the sciatic nerve. Also, the nerves at the base of the spine are vulnerable. The spinal cord stops growing in infancy, but the bones of the spine and rest of the body continue to grow. So the spinal cord ends near the top of the lumbar spine and yet a bunch of exposed nerve roots continue the journey towards the lower extremities. As a result of this, it becomes very easy for something to irritate one of these nerves.

In the case of piriformis syndrome, there is a muscle pressing on the sciatic nerve. The piriformis muscle crosses over the sciatic nerve. So if the piriformis muscle goes into spasm, then it will press on the sciatic nerve and create the same radiating pain that you'd get from a bone or disc pressing on the sciatic nerve. Muscles spasm for similar reasons – genetics, physical and emotional trauma, poor posture, diet and nutrition. We will get into the piriformis muscle and its functions in much more detail in chapter three. For now, it's simply important to understand that it too can cause sciatic pain.

In all of these situations, whether it is muscle or bone or disc pressing on the sciatic nerve, the key to healing is to change your habits. Those with chronic pain have an immediate incentive to seek solutions in changing their habits. Others may have pain every so often, but they too should change their habits to prevent the situation from continuing or growing worse. Perhaps you always seem to get injured in the same place or the same side. Maybe you've been to physical therapy that has been effectively only for the injury to recur again at a later date. Those who have had surgery should definitely examine their habits to create new, healthy patterns. Or perhaps you are not in pain but recognize these postural issues in yourself and know people in your life with sciatica. For all of us, it is vital to our health and healing that we consider the nature of the ways in which we move, get injured, and recover. How you live, move, and care for yourself will determine the quality of your life.

CHAPTER TWO: THE SCIATIC NERVE

Your nervous system runs the show. The central nervous system, comprised of the brain and spinal cord, receives and sends information through the peripheral nervous system, the nerves that radiate from the spinal cord through the rest of the body. Almost all of the body's nerves have to pass through holes in the spine to make their journeys. This makes the alignment of the spine key to a successfully functioning nervous system, as discussed.

Let's explore the nerve at the heart of this book – the sciatic nerve.

WHERE IS THE SCIATIC NERVE?

The sciatic nerve, also known as the ischiatic nerve, is the longest, widest single nerve in the body. It's the yellow nerve in the diagram on the left. At its largest point, it's as big around as an index finger. Take a moment to look at your index finger. It's pretty incredible to have a nerve this large moving through us. It deserves respect.

It begins in the lower back, and it is actually made up of five nerves that come out of the right and left hand side of the lower spine. You have a curve in your lower spine, and this area is referred

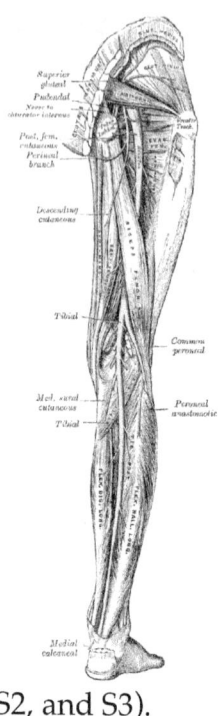

to as the lumbar spine. The lumbar spine includes five vertebrae (L1 – L5). Below the lumbar spine is the sacrum. The sacrum also consists of five vertebrae (S1 – S5). However these sacral vertebrae begin as unfused (like the rest of the spine), and then once we are standing and walking they fuse together making more of a plate. The nerves that make up the sciatic nerve come out of the bottom two lumber vertebrae (L4 and L5 and the top three sacral vertebrae S1, S2, and S3).

These five nerves come together out of L4, L5, S1, S2, and S3 to form two nerves, the tibial and the peroneal. These two nerves are incased in one sheath and together make the sciatic nerve. From the lower back, the sciatic nerve runs through the buttock and extends all the way down the back of the leg to the toes. At the back of the knee those two nerves, the tibial and peroneal, divide. You can see this in the diagram above. The peroneal travels sideways (laterally) along the outside of the knee to the upper foot. The tibial continues to travel downward to the feet, and it innervates the heel and sole of the foot.

Illustration: Gray's Anatomy

WHAT DOES THE SCIATIC NERVE DO?

With a nod to the above section, the sciatic nerve helps attach our torso to our legs. Specifically, it connects the spinal cord with the outside of the thigh, the hamstring muscles in the back of the thighs, and muscles in the lower leg and feet. More than physically connecting the legs to the body, the current of the sciatic nerve essentially connects your legs to your brain.

As a nerve, it is the electric current that makes the muscles work. It also transmits back to the brain what you feel in the leg. Simply put, the sciatic nerve supplies sensation and strength to the leg. This means that we need the current of the sciatic nerve to be running cleanly for us to use our legs well. It also provides the reflexes of the leg. Your reactions, feelings, movements in the legs all come from the sciatic nerve as it communicates with the brain. If you have a bad connection from the battery of the car to the headlight, then the headlight wouldn't work. These connections, like the sciatic nerve, keep us running.

When you are suffering from sciatic pain, it means that the nerve isn't running cleanly through the body. It is being impinged. Thus, in addition to the pain, you are also not getting clear messages from the brain to the leg and back again. You aren't using your incredibly powerful legs in an optimal way. Beyond the pain, sciatica is debilitating for your physical movement. We'll discuss this in more detail in chapter six.

WHAT IS THE SCIATIC NERVE'S RELATION TO THE PIRIFORMIS MUSCLE?

So those five nerves come together out of L4, L5, S1, S2, and S3 to make the sciatic nerve. They come together right on the front of the piriformis muscle. Basically the sciatic nerve is born at the piriformis muscle. But things can get even closer between the sciatic nerve and the piriformis. Remember how the sciatic nerve is actually two nerves – tibial and peroneal – that live in one sheath until they split at the back of the knee. In about 15% of the population, these two nerves split before they join up, so to speak. The peroneal segment will pass through the piriformis while the tibial runs in front of it, and then they will join up together to form the sciatic nerve. For some, this will never be an issue. But if the piriformis goes into spasm, then those individuals will feel sciatic pain. Because the peroneal segment is going through that muscle, there's no real "cure" for that, only a management of the pain by calming down the piriformis. Obviously the piriformis is intimately connected to the sciatic nerve; so let's take a closer look at this important muscle.

CHAPTER THREE:
THE PIRIFORMIS MUSCLE

Now we'll give the piriformis muscle the attention that it is due as a player in sciatica.

WHERE IS THE PIRIFORMIS MUSCLE?

The piriformis muscle is a flat, pyramidal shaped

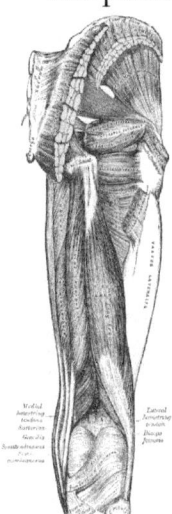

muscle. It's in red in the diagram on the left. One end of the piriformis connects to the sacrum. Again, this is the bottom portion of the spine where the vertebrae gradually become fused. The piriformis connects to the anterior sacrum (the front). From there, the piriformis muscle passes through the pelvis and then goes out via the greater sciatic foramen (opening). This is an opening in the pelvis that allows the sciatic nerve and the piriformis to travel from the spine to attach to the legs. As they make their journey through the pelvis, the sciatic nerve runs under the piriformis (and sometimes through the piriformis as discussed before). Obviously, with this close contact, the piriformis muscle can squeeze and irritate the sciatic nerve in this area. The other end of the piriformis connects to the greater trochanter, which is the bump on the

Illustation: Gray's Anatomy

outside of your thighbone (femur). You can feel this bump on the outside of the body if you dig in deep enough on the outer leg at the top.

WHAT DOES THE PIRIFORMIS MUSCLE DO?

The piriformis muscle is one of the external rotators of the hip and leg. External rotation is when you turn your leg out, away from the center of the body. Think ballerina or Charlie Chaplin. Also, the piriformis helps in abduction (moving the leg away from the body) when your hip is flexed (eg, when you draw your knee in towards your chest, something we do on a small scale every time we take a step). So if you wanted to have a seat cross-legged on the floor, you would use external rotation, hip flexion and abduction. Anyone who has suffered any of these symptoms knows that getting out of a car is no fun. Getting out of the car is a very common use of the piriformis muscle – you lift the leg (flexion), turn it out (external rotation), and move it away from the body (abduction). If you have sciatica or piriformis syndrome, you would probably feel it here. The piriformis muscle is working in fully glory!

The piriformis not only helps you to do these everyday actions but also stabilizes the hip joint while you do them. As discussed, the piriformis attaches at the greater trochanter (outside of the big thigh bone) and the anterior sacrum (inside the lowest part of the spine). Where your sacrum meets your pelvis, you have a sacroiliac joint (SI joint) that essentially creates the singular pelvis by connecting the two hip bones to either side of the sacrum. There are two tracks or grooves that allow for a tiny bit of movement within your SI joint. This allows for a stable yet moveable pelvis provided each piriformis (right and left) is equal in balance and tone. When one or both of the piriformis muscles are short or tight, it inhibits the SI joint on that side leading towards a host of problems that include sciatica and piriformis syndrome.

Further, the piriformis' tone and balance affects the performance of the deep gluteus muscles in many actions like moving the leg away from the body and rotating it in/out. We have three gluteal muscles – the big one (gluteus maximus) and two deeper glutes (minimus and medius). It's these deeper glutes that have a close relationship with the piriformis; they lie underneath it. They both abduct the leg (move it away from the body) and rotate it (internally and externally). If the piriformis muscle isn't working well, then the deep gluteal muscles underneath it can't fully execute their actions either. Your leg movements will accordingly be compromised.

The piriformis, this tiny muscle, affects the movements of your legs, hips, and spine, not to mention the health of your sciatic nerve. The tone and balance of your piriformis (on each side) is tremendously important to the body and your movement. One reason we lose tone in the piriformis is bad posture. A large majority of people stand and walk with their feet turned out (again, shortening the back body). Anatomical neutral, which would hopefully be our default posture, has the feet parallel. This gets to the basic design of the body and our posture, which we'll discuss

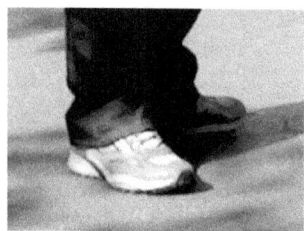 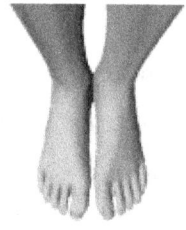

throughout. The shin bones are designed to be parallel and move straight up from parallel feet that stand fairly close together. The leg bones above the knee angle out to join the torso at the hip. This parallel stance of the feet creates the ideal resting position for the piriformis. You can feel this when standing. With the feet parallel the buttocks can be broad and untucked more easily. If the feet are turned out the piriformis is automatically shortened into a contracted state. If this is you natural posture and walking pattern your piriformis is slightly contracted 24/7, which compromises the movement of the legs, hips, and spine.

Finally, the piriformis is also one of only two muscles connecting the upper and lower body. The Psoas is the other one, and we'll discuss it next. Again, like the sciatic nerve, the connection aspect is a big deal. We need these connectors to be physically healthy for us to move well but also for us to feel grounded and stable as we move through the world.

In chapter 6, we'll look at piriformis syndrome and what happens when the muscle spasms. Next we'll address how the piriformis and psoas work together for our physical and emotional health.

CHAPTER FOUR:
THE PSOAS AND PIRIFORMIS

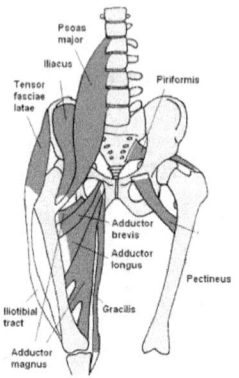

The psoas is the topic of the first book in our ebook series. It has come up in this book a few times already because of its importance. Let's explore it more with relation to the piriformis and sciatica.

WHAT IS THE PSOAS?

First, a quick review of the psoas (or an introduction if you haven't read our psoas ebook). In our opinion, the psoas is the most important muscle in the body. It is the main hip flexor. As mentioned, flexing is when we draw the leg closer to the chest. We do this action on a small scale each time we step the foot out in front of us. Therefore, the psoas is the main muscle for walking.

The psoas is also the main muscle for trauma. Anytime you are afraid, you flex. Notice what happens when you're startled or fearful, you flinch and flex. That's the nature of the beast. You're going to play possum (play dead) or you're going to fight or you're going to run. All of these three actions involve flexion, a shortening of the body. When you play dead, you curl up and the psoas draws the knees in to the chest. When you fight, you crouch, and the psoas helps you get small. When you run, you take your feet in front of you and the psoas moves them forward. When the fear responses kicks in, the psoas goes into action.

There is nothing wrong with the fear response. It's a natural part of being a human being! However, issues arise when that fear response doesn't go away. If we don't release that flexion, then your psoas becomes tight…and that continued tightness communicates to your brain and nervous system you're in danger. Basically you stay stuck in fight-or-flight. This happens to many of us whether we're stuck in daily anxiety or experiencing post-traumatic stress after a specific incident. Thus releasing the psoas is an extremely important piece of emotional health and also physical health. Releasing the psoas also helps the health of the piriformis, as the two are inseparable partners in the dance of the moving body. Let's look more at how these two muscles work together.

HOW DO THE PSOAS AND THE PIRIFORMIS WORK TOGETHER?

The psoas and piriformis are the only two muscles that connect the legs to the spine. They work like a stirrup, providing a downward pull on the sacrum (the bottom of your spine). The psoas pulls from the front and the piriformis pulls from the back. They essentially strap the upper and lower body together.

The psoas and piriformis took on this important role when we stood up! As quadrupeds the weight of the spine falls easily into both the arms and the legs. When stand upright, we use the hamstring and the now uber-important gluteus maximus, and the psoas and piriformis are working to hold us up in a balanced way. These two muscles while not necessarily dormant in the quadruped are now called on constantly to hold us up successfully.

As with all muscles, we want tone in the psoas and piriformis. Strong enough to move us but not overly contracted or tight. Moreover, because they work together, we need a balance between these two muscles. In fact, the tone and balance of these two muscles goes a long way to determining the successful upright posture.

WHAT DOES THIS HAVE TO DO WITH SCIATICA?

As we'll keep shouting from the rooftops, a good upright posture will prevent (and heal) sciatica. In terms of the psoas and piriformis, this requires them being balanced as stirrups on the sacrum. Again, this means not too contracted. The psoas and piriformis require a certain amount of tone to stay in place. However, they do not want to place themselves or hold themselves in position. This action would require over contracting and tightening you up and pulling you out of that good upright posture. Instead, the psoas and piriformis depend on a holy trinity of muscle groups to keep them in the right place. It is the tone of the inner thighs, pelvic floor, and abdominals that keeps the psoas and piriformis aligned. If these three groups are toned, then your psoas and piriformis are going to live in perfect alignment. Now because many of us do not use our inner thighs, pelvic floor and abdominals successfully, we tend to be weak in these areas…and thus over working our psoas and piriformis. This pulls us out of alignment. (And with a nod to the emotional state, this over working sends a message to our nervous system and brain to be in fight-or-flight.) So for many reasons, we will be providing exercises at the end of the book to both release our psoas and piriformis and will be providing exercises in our following ebook on the spine to strengthen the holy trinity of inner thighs, pelvic floor, and abdominals.

For now, let's round out the cast of characters in sciatica by exploring the lumbar spine and pelvis – the areas of origin for the sciatic nerve.

CHAPTER FIVE:
THE PELVIS AND THE LUMBAR SPINE

As we've seen, the sciatic nerve originates in the lumbar and sacral regions of the spine and then moves through an opening in the pelvis as it travels to our legs. This means that a toned and well-aligned spine and pelvis create an open, spacious environment for the sciatic nerve. Let's look at that more closely.

HOW DO THE PELVIS
AND SPINE FIT INTO THIS?

As your spine goes you go. Really, the health and alignment of your spine influence the health and alignment of your entire body.

The spine has four curves – two in and two out. We've discussed the bottom two already – lumbar and sacrum. But let's put the whole picture together. You have your cervical spine in your neck, which curves in. Then you have the thoracic spine around your chest (your ribcage), which curves out. Then you have lumbar, which curves in. Finally you have the sacrum, which curves out.

The lumbar vertebrae are the biggest and strongest. This makes sense intuitively. You can feel that this is your center of gravity. There are many important joints in this area of the body. However, three are of particular importance. One is the lumbosacral where the lumbar meets the sacrum, as the name implies. The other two are the iliofemoral where your femurs (thigh bones) meet the pelvis. The relationship of these joints affect the proper placement of your pelvis and this determines everything that happens above and below.

WHAT DOES THIS HAVE TO DO WITH SCIATICA?

Having the correct, natural curves to the spine is paramount. Or to put it bluntly – tucking the pelvis is death! As we've discussed, there is an aesthetic and cultural move towards tucking our pelvis under. This is not a natural position. We are supposed to have a curve in our lower back, the lumber spine.

We're also supposed to have a curve in the cervical spine, the neck. In fact, the cervical spine and lumbar spine are mirror images of each other. This means that the lower back and the neck are shaped in the same ways. They are designed to have the exact same degree of curve. In addition to seeing a lot of pelvic tucking (eliminating the lumbar curve) in our culture, we also see a lot of pushing the head forward (flattening the cervical curve). In our work at the walking program, the forward head posture is the most common postural misalignment we see. You can imagine how the head forward and pelvic tucking have developed together in our culture. Basically we're moving our heads towards our computers or TV's, while we sink into chairs and couches.

Unfortunately, this pushing forward of the head and tucking of the pelvic is not a good situation for the sciatic nerve and the piriformis muscle. It creates a tight, cramped space and also compromises the muscle tone of the lower back. We need this natural, correct curve in at L4 and L5 (the 4th and 5th vertebrae of the lumbar). This shape allows for good muscle tone and keeps the sacrum in the right place (curving out). Moreover, it creates for optimum space so the sciatic nerve can flow freely and the piriformis muscle will be naturally long and easy.

We'll talk more about the posture and how to correct it in chapter seven. For now, let's dive deeper into what sciatica actually is in terms of a diagnosed condition.

CHAPTER SIX:
SCIATICA AND PIRIFORMIS SYNDROME

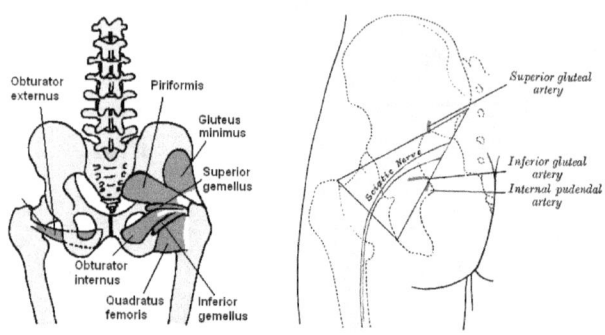

We've got the cast of characters in place. Let's get into more details about the star of the show - sciatica.

WHAT IS SCIATICA?

The clinical diagnosis of sciatica is referred to as a radiculopathy, which means nerve pain that originates in the spine. The vertebrae of our spine line up in a column (with those four curves we've discussed). Between each vertebra is a disc filled with fluid. Sometimes a disc protrudes from its normal position in the vertebral column. When the disc slips out of alignment, it pushes up against the nerve root in the lower back. This nerve root forms part of the sciatic nerve. And the pain begins. Imagine, you have a water balloon in your hands and a string is hanging right behind it. If you squeeze the balloon, it squishes out and touches the string. That hurts when the string is the root of your sciatic nerve.

An important thing to consider is that sciatica is the symptom of the problem — of something compressing or irritating the nerve roots that comprise the sciatic nerve. It is not a medical disorder in and of itself. Obviously it's important to figure out why you are having the pain, why your disc is protruding. The exercises we give can help you relieve it, but it's still good to understand what has happened inside your body.

Sciatica occurs most frequently in people between 30 and 50 years of age. Often a particular event or injury does not cause sciatica, but rather it tends to develop as a result of general wear and tear on the structures of the lower spine. We've talked about why discs could slip – genetics, physical and emotional trauma, diet and nutrition, and poor posture. Let's examine the issue with more detail. Common causes of sciatica include the following low back conditions: spinal disc herniation, degenerative disc disease, spinal stenosis, spondylolysis, tumors and pregnancy. Before we share with you a basic description of these issues we want to put out a thought that would be useful for everyone. When you get injured and go to the doctor with these kinds of issues they will often send you for an MRI. MRIs are amazing tool, but they only give you a snapshot of that given moment. What would the film have shown a year prior? We believe that if it is at all possible people should have MRIs done at some time so that there is a baseline to compare future test too. The more information we have the more likely we will negotiate successful outcomes to our body's troubles. On to causes of sciatica pain:

- Spinal disc herniation, often referred to as a "slipped disc", is a condition in which a fissure in the outer ring of an intervertebral disc lets the soft middle seep out. Imagine that water balloon again (your disc), but let's fill it with jelly. A fissure in the outer layer would allow that jelly to begin leaking out. Discs almost always slip to the side (leak out the side) due to strong ligaments lining the back of the spine. Most herniations in the lower back happen between the fourth and fifth lumbar vertebrae or between the fifth lumbar vertebrae and the sacrum. As we know, this is right where the sciatic nerve originates.

- Degenerative disc disease is not really a disease but a term used to describe the normal changes in the spinal column as you age. Between each vertebra there is a soft cushion that acts as a shock absorber for the spine, allowing it to flex, bend, and twist. Poor posture and bad movement patterns can lead to this problem which in turn can lead to a host of other problems like sciatica.

- Spinal Stenosis is a narrowing of the spine occurring most often in the neck or lower back. This narrowing can put pressure on the spinal cord or spinal nerves at the level of compression. Spinal stenosis is commonly thought to be caused by age-related changes in the spine. As always we feel that poor mechanics and conditioned patterns have more to due with the body's breakdown that anything else. In severe cases of spinal stenosis, doctors perform surgery to create additional space for the spinal cord or nerves.

- Spondylolysis and Spondylolisthesis-Spondylolysis results from a weakness in a section of the vertebra called the pars interarticularis, the thin piece of bone that connects the upper and lower segments of the facet joints. Facet joints link together the upper and lower joints of the vertebrae to form a working unit that permits movement of the spine. The pars interarticularis is found in the posterior (back) of the vertebra. Spondylolysis occurs when there is a fracture of the pars portion of the vertebra. Spondylolisthesis occurs when the vertebra shifts forward due to instability from the pars defect. Again we feel that this type of injury is most commonly caused by conditioned patterns and habits. When the structural alignment of the spine is not working optimally, the environment for stress fractures increases exponentially

- Tumors can develop in the body that directly affect the spine and nerves creating all of the same symptoms commonly associated with sciatica.

- Pregnancy causes the uterus to grow and drop, which can cause it to press directly onto the sciatic nerve causing terrible discomfort often for long portions of pregnancy. This is often alleviated post partum. However, the movement habits we acquire during pregnancy have a way of sticking around and can cause us problems as we continue through life.

Again, much of this comes back to the posture. Herniation, degeneration, stenosis, and spondylolisthesis – all of these can happen as a result of poor posture. The good news is that if your body is well aligned and your muscles are well toned, then there is no reason why any of those things are going to happen. Don't accept that everybody degenerates and loses their posture and becomes shorter. There is no reason for a bony degeneration to happen. The correct curve of the lumbar spine will determine how the sciatic nerve passes through to get to the leg.

We've discussed the general need for the curves in the back to create a healthy, spacious environment for the sciatic nerve. The iliofemoral ligament also plays a role. Ligaments connect bone to bone. The iliofemoral ligament is the strongest ligament in the body. It connects the femur (thighbone) to the ilium (pelvis). When this ligament has its proper tone, the leg and the pelvis are really nicely connected and alignment is achievable. However, once again, as a result of the thighs falling forward in most peoples' posture (short back body, long front body), the iliofemoral ligament is overly stretched. This compromises the stability of the pelvis and, again, the flow of the sciatic nerve.

WHAT IS PIRIFORMIS SYNDROME?

As discussed, piriformis syndrome also causes sciatic pain. Sometimes sciatica from a slipped disc is referred to as "true" sciatica. But anyone who has experienced sciatic pain from piriformis syndrome will assure you that her pain is true as well. With piriformis syndrome, sciatic pain develops because your piriformis muscle is rubbing on the sciatic nerve and irritating it.

To review, the tibial and peroneal nerves form the sciatic nerve. These nerves come out of the lumbar spine and the sacrum and meet in front of the piriformis to form the sciatic nerve. (Again, for a small number of us the peroneal passes through the piriformis.) When the piriformis muscle goes into spasm it presses against the sciatic nerve. That is piriformis syndrome. In order to relieve the sciatic pain, you'll need to release the piriformis muscle.

The piriformis muscle could go into spasm for several reasons. Very often a sedentary lifestyle leads to problems with the piriformis as sitting for long periods, especially at desks that are not ergonomically inclined, tends to irritate the muscles and nerves. Flying a lot, or driving long distances is a classic way to encourage and maintain these problems. It can be as simple as carrying a wallet in your back pocket, or as we have referred to over and over again, standing or walking with your feet turned out put the muscles into an unnatural position at all times. Further, women encounter piriformis syndrome 6 times more often than men simply because of the shape of their pelvis.

Sciatic pain is a symptom, a very painful symptom of either bony alignment issues or piriformis syndrome. Healing can't begin without a correct diagnosis. From a diagnostic standpoint it is a simple yet very important distinction between whether you have sciatica or piriformis syndrome. If the pain is in the lower back radiating down, it is sciatica. If the pain begins in your butt and moves down from there, you have piriformis syndrome.

However, in doing the work to alleviate the pain through improved posture and strengthening/releasing exercise, you will be helping the problem of misalignment of the spine as well as the tension of the piriformis.

CHAPTER SEVEN – POSTURE

Good alignment is the best thing you can give yourself to avoid sciatica. It's preventative medicine – good posture prevents bony degeneration, good posture prevents muscle degeneration, good posture prevents sciatica. But good posture can also address sciatica once it's started. It can alleviate this painful symptom and often its causes as well.

HOW DO WE LEARN POSTURE?

Some of us learned basic anatomy in school, but we didn't learn functional movements, nor did we practice them. Long gone are the deportment classes where you walked with a block on your head. When I tell people that we teach walking they respond with surprise – don't we know how to walk? Well, when you have a little baby you're going to teach her how to use a fork, you're going to teach him how to zip up his pants. The day they stand up to walk you simply say, "Yaaaay!" and then leave them to their own devices. Usually we learn our walking and other functional movements by imitation. We tend to imitate those we bond with, usually our parents – but also grandparents, babysitters, aunts and uncles. Our first movements are always about who was closest to us. So we essentially walk how our parents walk. I have seen instances of kids needing occupational therapy because their father is gimpy and the kid starts walking with that kind of limp.

This means that if you have a mother who has sciatica and you love your mother and walk like her, you're likely to have sciatica later in life. The flip side is if you are a mother with sciatica and you have a two-year-old daughter, you have incentive to not only get out of your pain but also spare your daughter a lifetime of your unhealthy conditioned patterns that she'll learn.

From our perspective, if you have good posture then everything is good. You're going to breathe well; you're going to have good blood flow; you're going to have good nervous energy; you're going to be happier about life. No joke. You'll probably love your dog more. Everything works when you have good posture. If you stand well, you are going to minimize the wear and tear on the body. You'll minimize the likelihood of chronic injuries and the likelihood of poor conditioned patterns. You won't do as much compensating for injuries or imbalanced muscles. You'll be more fully evolved!

WHAT IS NOT SO GOOD POSTURE?

Let's explore this short in the back, long in the front posture we've been discussing. The overwhelming majority of people fall into this postural category -- essentially splayed open.

If you think about the way most people are standing, their feet turn out a little bit, their stance is a little wide, their thighs sink forward, their pelvis is tucked under, their shoulders fall backwards and their neck is short, their chin is elevated, their lower back is short and their belly is somewhat stuck out. And that is modern man or woman. That is modern person. That is, I would say, 90% of the people we see at The FitzGordon Core Walking Program.

Let's look again at the diagram we shared before:

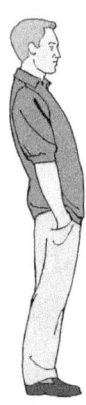

Illustation: Frank Morris

Now that you have some knowledge of the players in the situation of sciatica, you can see more how this posture would create problems. You can see how there's a sinking in the lower back (lumbar spine and sacrum) where the sciatic nerve begins to form. You can see how bony degeneration in these regions would lead to a slipped disc that could press into the origination of the sciatic nerve. Next, the sciatic nerve flows under (and perhaps through) the piriformis. You can see how the short back body and long front body would lead to weaknesses in the abdominals and inner thighs, which in turn requires the psoas and piriformis to over work to stay in the proper position. With this over-contracting comes potential for tension and the muscle spasms of piriformis syndrome. Next the sciatic nerve travels through the pelvis to the leg. You can see how the tucking of the pelvis and overstretching of the iliofemural ligament would put the pelvis in the improper place further compromising the path of the sciatic nerve. There are many opportunities in this common posture to inhibit the healthy flow of the sciatic nerve.

WHAT IS GOOD POSTURE?

Let's take a look at what good posture would mean.

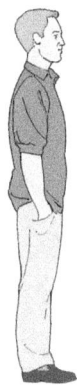

Illustation: Frank Morris

Here's a diagram where everything is stacked well.

There are four curves in the spine. The lumbar curve mirrors the cervical curve. There's lift and order to the vertebrae, keeping the discs in place. This stance requires tone in the abdominals, inner thighs and even the pelvic floor. In turn, these muscle groups allow the psoas and piriformis to reside in their proper place. The proper position of the pelvis allows for a toned but not overstretched iliofemural ligament. The entire pathway for the sciatic nerve is open and clear. It's really a beautiful thing.

So how do you stand this way?

- Untuck your pelvis and release your butt. The big butt muscles (gluteus maximus) should be completely turned off when standing.

- Let your thigh bones fall backwards under the pelvis. There is a side seam in most pants. That seam should be perpendicular to the floor

- Let the upper body hinge forward as the thighs go back. Think literally of a hinge with the pelvis as the pin.

- From the front, lower the bottom of the rib cage and the chin slightly allowing the middle rather than the upper back to round and broaden

- Lift the head slightly from the back of the

neck. Gaze straight ahead keeping the eye sockets level.

Now because of our conditioned pattern to be short in the back and long in the front, standing this way can feel really strange at first. You will feel like you're sticking your butt way out because you're used to tucking it under. You'll feel like you're rounding your shoulders because you're used to throwing them back to compensate for the collapsed chest. You won't recognize how to open up the back of the rib cage or how to soften the front of the rib cage. In short, you'll feel a bit like an ape…or so clients have told us.

But if you work with the exercises in this book and the walking program, you can change your patterns. You can learn the how and why of your movements and change them from a very deep place. Once you understand what it means to have a conditioned pattern, a pattern that is not of your choosing, you can choose a new pattern. You can learn how to truly stand on your own two feet.

CHAPTER EIGHT - STRETCH VS. RELIEF

Now that we've straightened up our posture, let's go back to the muscles and how to help them.

As a quick review - for the nervous system to work at its peak the bones have to be well aligned. And the bones can only be well aligned if the muscles are properly toned. So you have to tone the muscles to allow for the nervous energy to flow.

We've talked about muscle posture and tone. But have you noticed an absence of everyone's favorite advice around helping pain and muscles…stretch! Well, that's because stretching isn't always the solution. If I had to guess, you have tried to stretch your way out of whatever problem you are having for a long time. There is a point where you look at your system, situation and condition and say that stretching is not the answer. Unfortunately, for the most part, when you go to doctors with sciatica and piriformis syndrome, they first tell you to stretch and then tell you to have surgery. We need to figure out a way out of that.

One solution is to have a more educated look at your muscles. A lot of muscles are tight and a lot of muscles are full of tension. And you can be both; you can be tight and full of tension. A muscle that is tight can very often be stretched open. However, a muscle that is full of tension (carrying physical and emotional tension) must be released out of that tension before it can be healed and repaired.

WAIT! STRETCHING ISN'T THE ANSWER?!?

The major difference that we're presenting here is that stretching is not necessarily the answer. There are plenty of stretches in the upcoming exercises but we're emphasizing more of the release work – the idea of letting go, the idea of changing conditioned patterns, not by doing more but by doing less and letting go.

Especially when you're talking about a muscle in spasm like the piriformis or an overly tight or tense muscle like the psoas. Stretching is a meaningless thing because the muscle is in spasm or stuck in contraction. In these cases, a focus on release will be much more productive.

It gets into this question of stretch versus release. What is the best approach to a muscle - is it the best approach to stretch a muscle to bring it relief from its tension or is it the best approach to release a muscle? Stretching the piriformis is about making a muscle longer. Releasing the piriformis is taking a muscle that is over worked and letting it not work; you change its relationship to life.

WILL I EVER WANT TO STRETCH MUSCLES LIKE THE PIRIFORMIS AND PSOAS?

You'll have to explore for yourself. See what brings you relief. Truthfully you can't really stretch a muscle that is filled with tension. You'll stretch and stretch, but nothing will change. Have you ever had this experience? You'll need to experiment with the release exercises and see if this brings relief. From there perhaps you can move into stretching to lengthen the healthy, alive muscle. Again, the exercises will let you play with both to see what works better for you and in what order. You'll start to see changes and understand your body in a whole new way. You'll feel agency over your person. You'll begin to truly inhabit yourself.

CHAPTER NINE:
OPTIONS AND EXERCISES

First, let's review some of the options you have when dealing with sciatica. These are very brief introductions to the options. Please do much more research on your own if you're considering one of these.

1. Change your posture and learn how to walk (www.fitzgordonmethod.com) – Obviously, this is where we recommend that you start. You can make huge changes in your physical and emotional health by following the advice in this book, doing the exercises in this and other books, and working with the FitzGordon Core Walking Program. This requires you doing work for yourself to heal yourself. Though it takes times and dedication, it is incredibly empowering to take charge of your body and health.

2. Network Spinal Analysis – Also known as Network Chiropractic, this method was founded and developed by Dr. Donny Epstein and was an outgrowth of his original education as a chiropractor. Network Spinal Analysis, through specific low force touches to the spine, assists in developing new

strategies to dissipate tension from the spine and nerves. This allows you to connect with your body's natural rhythms and experience greater well-being.

3. Rolfing and/or Hellerwork – These are systems that realign or reorganize the body through working on the connective tissue or fascia. Essentially you are wearing a giant stocking inside called fascia. It connects and supports your muscles, bones, nerves and organs. With Rolfing or Hellerwork, a therapist works on this connective tissue. It feels like a very (VERY!) deep massage and can realign the body, returning you to healthy patterns and alleviating pain. I am so enamored of rolfing that I named my daughter Ida after its founder Ida Rolf.

4. Applied Kinesiology (AK) – This is a form of diagnosis using muscle testing as a primary feedback mechanism to examine how a person's body is functioning. When properly applied, the outcome of an AK diagnosis will determine the best form of therapy for the patient. Since AK draws together the core elements of many complementary therapies, it provides an interdisciplinary approach to health care. In general, the applied kinesiologist

finds a muscle that tests weak and then attempts to determine why that muscle is not functioning properly. The practitioner will then evaluate and apply therapy that will best eliminate the muscle weakness and help the patient. Therapies utilized can include specific joint manipulation or mobilization, various myofascial therapies, cranial techniques, meridian therapy, clinical nutrition, dietary management and various reflex procedures.

5. Acupuncture – A form of Traditional Chinese Medicine, acupuncture recognizes that we have energy flowing through our bodies and it gets stuck due to tension or patterns or injuries. It is this stuck energy that leads to disease or chronic pain. The provider will place (very small) needles on pressure points. Sometimes the needle is placed directly on the site of injury or tension. Other times it is placed in the corresponding pressure point. For example, tension in the left leg might require needles in the right arm. This system works well with our idea that often we need not stretching but releasing tension from areas of the body. We like to think that anything that has been around for 3000 years must have something going for it.

Surgery – In our opinion, this would be your last resort. Simply put, it is a big deal to open up the body and there is no guarantee of success. That said, having had three knee surgeries due to poor alignment and execution in my yoga practice, I understand that when necessary surgery can be useful and effective. But as always it is our post surgery routines and rehab that will determine how well we heal. I had my last surgery in 1998 and haven't had a consequential injury since. But the truth is after my last surgery (you think I would have learned after the first one), I completely changed. My patterns no longer resemble the man of my youth. Please explore every option before taking the surgical plunge.

EXERCISES

Let's look at some basic releases and stretches that can help with sciatica and piriformis syndrome.

Release work is about letting go. This requires some hanging out in each pose for breathing and letting tension dissolve.

CONSTRUCTIVE REST POSITION (CRP)

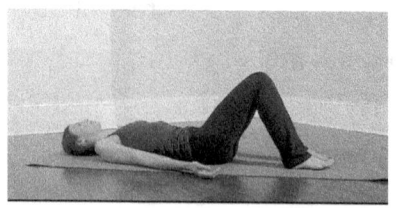

This is the main psoas release that we work with. It is a gravitational release of the psoas that allows the force of gravity to have its way with the contents of the trunk and the deep core.

- Lie on your back with your knees bent and your heels situated 12 to 16 inches away from your pelvis, in line with your sit bones.

- Tie a belt around the middle of the thighs. You want to be able to let go here and not have to think too much about the position of your legs.

- Then do nothing. Discomfort arises from conditioned muscular patterns. Try not to shift or move when unpleasant sensations arise.

- You are hoping to feel sensations that you can sit with, and if possible, allow them to pass.

- Try to do this for 30 minutes a day. If you have time, longer sessions are advisable, or do it twice a day.

Remember, you are not here to suffer. If sensations come up and you feel that you have to move, feel free to move, then come back to where you were and try again. It's possible that you'll do this exercise and not feel anything; it will still be good for you.

BLOCK LUNGES

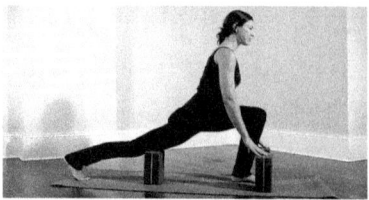

This is a release of both the quadriceps and the psoas. Sometimes the quadriceps muscles are so tight, there is no getting to the psoas until we release the quads a bit. You'll need three blocks for this.

- Positioned on your hands and knees, step the right foot forward in between your hands. Use two blocks under your hands by your front foot.

- Place a third block underneath the quadriceps muscle of the back leg just above the knee, at the base of the thigh.

- Tuck the back toes and let the weight of the body fall onto the block. Do your best to keep the heel of the back foot pointing straight up toward the ceiling.

- The front leg and hip should not be under any strain. Feel free to make adjustments, turning the foot out or stepping the foot wider.

- You need to stay for 90 seconds to get the full benefits of this pose.

RECLINING COBBLER'S POSE

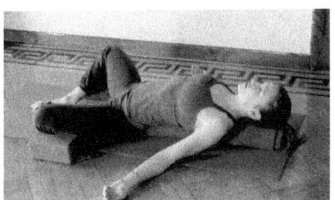

- Lay flat on your back with a blanket or towel rolled up, lengthwise under your spine. You could also place pillows under you. Your torso and head should feel supported. Make sure the head is extending with the spine and not dropping back.

- Bring the soles of the feet together as close to the hips as possible.

- Keeping the soles of the feet together, let the knees fall open to the side.

- Support the outer leg with blocks or blankets or pillows under the thighs.

- Let everything go as long as you feel supported in the shape.

- This puts the piriformis at rest, not allowing it to do anything.

- Try to stay for 10 – 20 minutes

ANKLE TO KNEE BACKWARDS

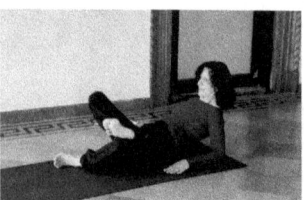 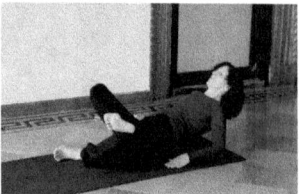

- Try and stack your shins on top of one another, right shin on top to begin.

- Flex the feet strongly and try to avoid letting the ankle collapse into the leg underneath it.

- Belt your legs at wherever they end up. Put the belt around the feet and knees. Don't make the belt tighter trying to deepen the pose. You just want to make it tight enough so that your top knee can't lift up and out of the shape.

- If you look down between your legs there should be a triangle of open space, the leg should be right on top of one another. Sit evenly on both sit bones.

- Slowly and easily begin to move backwards walking the hands behind you. Make sure not to tuck your pelvis under to move back. If anything stick your butt out a little.

- This is very likely to be an extreme stretch of the hip flexors and the top of the thigh. Try sighing to let the top knee release.

- If you can go onto your forearms give that a

shot. BUT, don't tuck the pelvis under and don't go deeper just to do it. Find the place of tension and hang out there.

- Change and put the other shin on top.

ANKLE OVER KNEE AT WALL

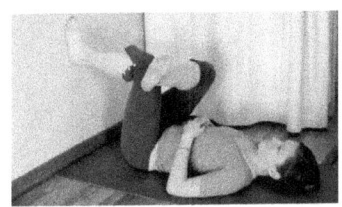

- Lay flat on your back with your knees bent and your toes at the base of a wall.

- Cross the right ankle over the left knee. Flex the right foot.

- Keep your lower back naturally arched a tiny bit off of the floor.

- Draw the left knee towards your chest and place your left foot on the wall

- Try your best to keep your right shin parallel to the chest while still reaching your tailbone down to the floor and your shoulders relaxed down on the floor.

- Stay for as long as fifteen minutes.

- Change sides.

TIGHT HIP RELEASE

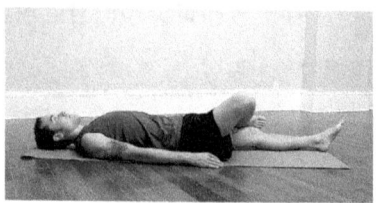

This is a passive release for extremely tight hips.

- Lie on your back with the legs straight out on the floor. Stabilize the trunk and bring the right foot up as high up on the left thigh as possible. If your right knee is lifted up higher than the ankle, this is a good release exercise for you.

- Allow the right knee to release toward the floor, keeping the trunk stable the entire time.

- Try to let the release come from both the inner and outer thigh as gravity takes the leg toward the floor.

- Stay for five minutes on each side if possible.

FROG BELLY

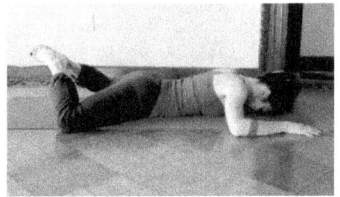

- Lay on your belly.

- Bend the knees out to the side and bring the feet together. They will likely be a foot or so off of the floor.

- Hang in there. This will likely be an intense stretch in the hip flexor but mainly it shuts piriformis off and lets it relax.

- You can try to bring your knees higher out to the side for a variation, or you can separate your feet about eight inches apart.

- Stay for a few minutes.

FOOT ON A BLOCK

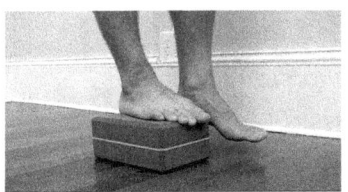 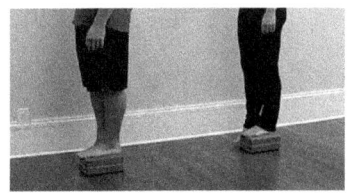

This is a gravitational release of the psoas…one that you can do on the street by dangling a foot off the curb while holding on to a lamppost.

- Place a block (or stack of large books) 8 to 10 inches from a wall.

- Step the left foot up on the block, allowing the right foot to hang down between the block and the wall. Place your right arm on the wall to help you stabilize the upper body.

- Keep the hips level and rotate the inner back thighs back and apart – stick out your butt a bit, and feel like you can let go from the base of the rib cage (the top of the psoas).

- Once you are comfortable with the leg hanging out of the hip, you can move the leg half an inch forward and back as slowly and steadily as possible. Half an inch is a very short distance.

- Let the leg dangle this way for 30 seconds or until the standing hip has done enough.

- Switch sides and tune in to which side is tighter. Do the second side for the same length of time that you did the first side.

- Repeat for a second time on the tighter side.

SOFT BALL UNDER SACRUM AND/OR NECK

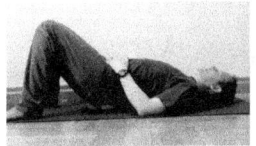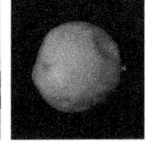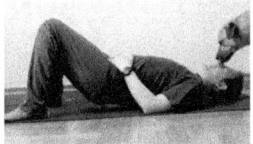

- You need a very soft and pliable ball for this exercise.
- Place the ball under your sacrum and relax onto it.
- You can roll around little bit but basically just try to hang out.
- After a few minutes (up to 15) deflate the ball a little bit and move it to the base of the head. Not under the neck, but at the place where the spine meet the cranium.
- Chill.

STRETCHS

As with the release, time is a part of the equation in stretches. You want to stay in each pose for many breaths and slow the breathing down. See if you can breath right into the area with sensation. Pay attention to the sensation – how does it change as you stay, do it have a color to it or a shape, is it localized or general. This kind of observation will help the body to open (shining a light on the issue lets the body relax) and help you to understand what is going on with your body. If you take yoga, you may recognize some of these.

SITTING ON A CHAIR, LEAN FORWARD WITH FLAT BACK

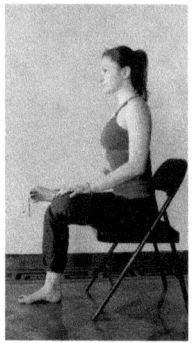 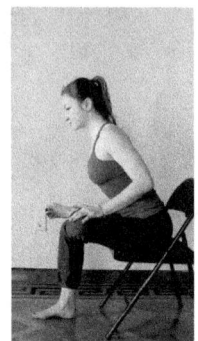

- Sit upright in a chair with a flat back.

- Cross the right ankle over the left knee. Flex the right foot (push through the heel).

- Begin to lean forward keeping the natural arches in the back (meaning don't round forward and collapse your chest).

- If the lower back begins to round backwards, stop. You have gone to far. Go back to a point where you can keep the curve in the lower back and breath here.

ANKLE OVER KNEE ON BACK

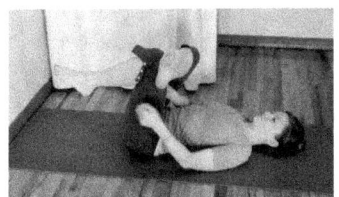 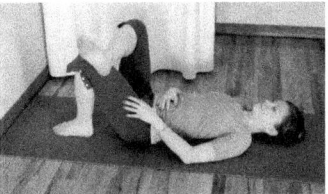

This is a great one to start with – you might recognize it from junior high gym class!

- Lay flat on your back.

- Bend your knees; bring your feet flat to the floor.

- Cross the right ankle over the left knee. Flex the right foot.

- Keep your lower back naturally arched a tiny bit off of the floor.

- Draw the left knee towards your chest and your right knee away from you. You can hold onto the back of your left thigh (left hand goes around the left leg; right hand goes between the legs).

- Try your best to keep your right shin parallel to the chest while still reaching your tailbone down to the floor and your shoulders relaxed down on the floor.

- Stay for many breaths, breathing

- Change sides

ANKLE TO KNEE FORWARD BEND

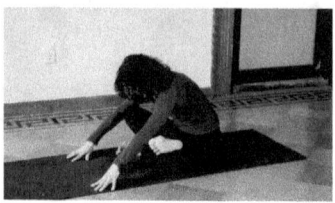 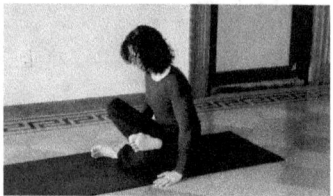

This stretch happens in two parts depending on what you feel in the first part.

- Sit with the legs straight out in front of you. Cross the right ankle over the left knee. Try to not to excessively round the back. Feel the natural curves in the spine. Life the chest and lean forward. If you feel this in your piriformis (side of the butt) this is as far as you'll go. Take deep breaths and then change sides. If you feel this in your hamstring (back of the leg) you will move onto the second stage.

- Keep your right ankle on top of your left knee and bend the left knee placing the left ankle below the right knee. (It's a deeper version than sitting "cross-legged".)

- Try and stack your shin on top of one another, right shin on top. The left shin should be hiding underneath the right shin.

- Stay even on both sit bones. Most people need to press their hands down, lift the butt up, and then place the butt down again taking the sit bone of the leg that's on top down to the floor first.

- Flex the feet strongly and try to avoid letting the top ankle collapse down into the leg that's below it.

- If you look down between your legs there should be a triangle of open space, the leg should be right on top of one another.

- Extend forward stretching deep into the piriformis. Breath.

- Do the other side.

STANDING PIGEON

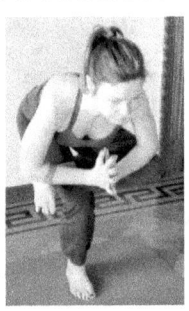 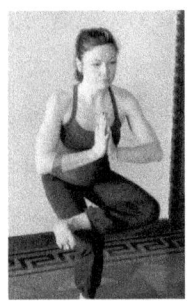

Stand with the feet hip distance apart and parallel.

- Cross the right ankle over the left knee. Flex the right foot strongly (push through the heel).

- Begin to squat. Think about lowering down backwards more than leaning forward. Stick the butt out.

- If you can bring the forearms onto the right shin, place them there and hold.

- Ideally the right shin is parallel to both the front of your mat and the floor.

- Breath.

- Change sides.

PIGEON

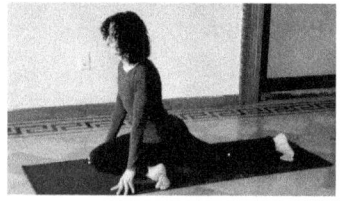 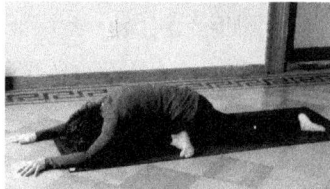

- Starting on your hands and knees slide your right knee towards your right wrist. Make sure that your right foot moves forward enough to get to the outside of the left thigh. If you fall onto the outside of your right hip, you may need to support that hip with a pillow or folded blanket.

- Slide the left leg straight back and make sure that the ankle is lined up with the knee and hip and that the foot is pointed straight.

- Walk the hands back alongside the hips and then try to and bring your hips towards square. (You will see that when the right leg is in front, the right hip pulls forward. Try to pull the right hip back and bring the left hip forward. You will probably feel more in your right hip as you do this.)

- Bow forward keeping the arms active and find the stretch deep in the right buttock. Take many breaths here.

- Change sides.

Butt Stretch

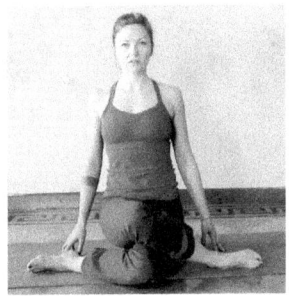

- You might want to sit up on a block or a few pillows or folded blankets (or towels) to begin this stretch.

- Come onto your hands and knees. Put your right knee in front of your left, both feet sticking out to the sides of you.

- Sit back between your feet onto your support.

- Try to keep the right knee on top of the left. For many of us it will lift and move to the right a bit. That's fine.

- Bow forward. If this seems relatively doable, lower the support. If that is also easy, sit your butt on the floor.

- Breathe.

- Change sides.

TWIST ON BACK

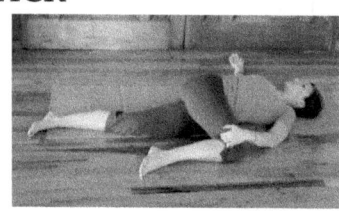

- Lay flat on your back.

- Draw the right knee into the chest and keep the left leg extending long on the floor.
  The left toes point straight up towards the ceiling.

- Begin to twist drawing the right knee across the left side of the body. The right knee can go over as much as possible, even reaching the floor if that work (or you could put a block or blanket or pillow under it).

- Let the left hand rest on the right thigh. Reach your right arm out to the right.

- Keep tone in the belly and look over the right shoulder. Slow down the breath and let the stretch happen.

- Change sides.

SQUATS

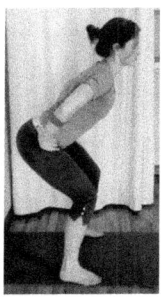

Stand up straight with feet shoulder's-width apart or slightly wider. Keep the feet as close to parallel as possible making sure to work equally on both sides. Feel free to hold onto a chair as you begin to explore this exercise

- Slowly and steadily bend your knees and flex your hips to lower your butt toward the floor. Don't let your knees move forward of the toes. You are trying to squat down backwards.

- Don't worry about how far down you can go at first. Work on maintained alignment and a pain free descent.

- Lower down to the best of your ability and hold for five breaths. Try to increase this over time to 25 breaths.

- An advanced variation is to isolate and engage your pelvic floor muscles while squatting. In this version you try to tone the levator ani (a thick muscle at the top of the pelvic floor. The pelvic floor consists of three layers, the sphincters, the perineum and the all important levator ani) for both lowering into the squat and lifting back up. This creates both eccentric and concentric contraction of deep muscles (Muscles work in a number of ways. They can engage and contract (concentric), engage and expand (eccentric), and engage without moving (isometric).) That can help ease the strain on the piriformis.

Give the stretch and release work a try. See which exercises are harder or easier. See how you feel after each one. Try to let the ego move out of the way and work from your wisdom. What does your body want to do? Your body knows how to heal itself. Work with it. Listen to it. Help you, help you!

WHAT ABOUT PLAIN OLD EXERCISE?

We are strong believers in exercise and think people should be exercising an hour a day. It's not about cardio though; it's about using the body and getting the muscles toned and balanced. As you've heard and read many times, find something that you enjoy. Find movement that interests you and challenges you and inspires you. If you're currently in pain, find exercise that works for you. Let go of expectations of what "working out" is supposed to be and follow your instincts. As your body changes, your interest in different exercise programs will change as well. Meet your body where it is and enjoy what you can do. Your body is an incredible machine. Exercising it daily helps you to appreciate and care for this vehicle.

ANYTHING ELSE? YES, HYDRATE!

Maybe drinking water doesn't count as an exercise? But hydration also has a huge connection to sciatica and piriformis syndrome and degenerative spines and bones and muscle tone. An interesting thought is from the time you're born you're drying up. You're here to dry out, degenerate. Ashes to ashes. We've heard that you're born you're 85% water, and when you die you're down to around 35%. It's a fascinating process. The quality of the bone and muscle tissue and blood and oxygen we pass, it is all connected to hydration…and posture and muscle tone. So part of your regular self-care routine should be to drink plenty of water and eat water-containing fruits and vegetables. Maybe this will be the easiest exercise we've given you!

CHAPTER TEN: CONCLUSION

You shouldn't live with the pain of sciatica and piriformis syndrome. You can change your body. We realize that it can feel overwhelming to consider that your current posture, your deeply engrained conditions, your current stretching exercises…none of it may be helping you and might even be hurting you. However, none of this work to bring relief has to be difficult. Learning to align your bones and free your muscles is a joyous process that brings ease and release. It's not about difficulty. It's about exploration and progress.

Your legs and lower body are what connect you to the earth. They ground you. They keep you stable and help you move through life, literally and figuratively. Helping your legs and lower body move in a fluid and pain-free way will impact your life on many dimensions. You will go forward in new and exciting ways. It is very worth the investment of time and energy to help free yourself from pain. Moreover, becoming more conscious and aware of how you move your body and improving that movement will help you become more aware across your entire life. You deserve this awareness of your life and fluidity of movement. Take advantage of living in your incredible body. Enjoy this amazing gift! Be well!

Acknowledgements

I have learned from so many people both in person and in print. Here is a short list of those who influenced this book.

Therese Bertherat, Genny Kapuler, Bonnie Bainbridge Cohen, Irene Dowd, John Friend, Sandra Jamrog, Bessel van der Kolk, Liz Koch, Peter Levine, Tom Myers, Jenny Otto, Ida Rolf, Lulu Sweigard.

And to the many students who have been patient with me on my path to learning. You have been my true teachers and my true guides.

Thanks as well to artists and Models:

Raina Passo, Beth Hyde, Frank Morris, Molly Fitzsimons, Jesse Kaminash,, Chris Marx,

Special thanks to Katie Malachuk.